Nature's Medicine: The Ultimate Homeopathic and Alternative Therapy Guide to Combating Common Problems and Stubborn Illnesses

Summary

The information on this eBook is intended to equip you with the knowledge you are so eager to get regarding diagnosing, prevention, treatment and cure of common health problems. However, you should consult a health physician to learn more about the health problem you are facing before you start taking herbal remedies, this is more important for pregnant women and individuals with an underlying health condition. Consulting a health physician before you start up on any herbal supplement program is a must to be on the safe side.

The book has an in-depth explanation of the health benefits you gain from using nature's medicine. All the herbs that you can use to boost your immune system to make it stronger and increase its effectiveness in fighting long term illness has also been well explained in chapter 5. In addition to the health benefits, the eBook also highlights the differences between conventional and herbal medicine, providing readers with the reasons they should take one and ignore the other.

Table of Contents

Summary 3

Introduction 5

Chapter 1: What Is Nature's Medicine 6

Chapter 2: How Nature's Medicine Works 9

Chapter 3: Most Common Natural Medicine for Men 12

Chapter 4: Nature's Medicine For Women 16

Chapter 5: Natures Medicine For Weight Loss 20

Chapter 6: Natures Medicine Remedies For Children 24

Chapter 7: Nature's Medicine /Modern Conventional Techniques 31

Chapter 8: 4 Ways To Relive Pain Using Natural Medicine 37

Chapter 9: Using Natural Medicine To Boost Your Immune System 42

Chapter 10: Heath Benefits Of Natural Medicine 52

Conclusion 58

Introduction

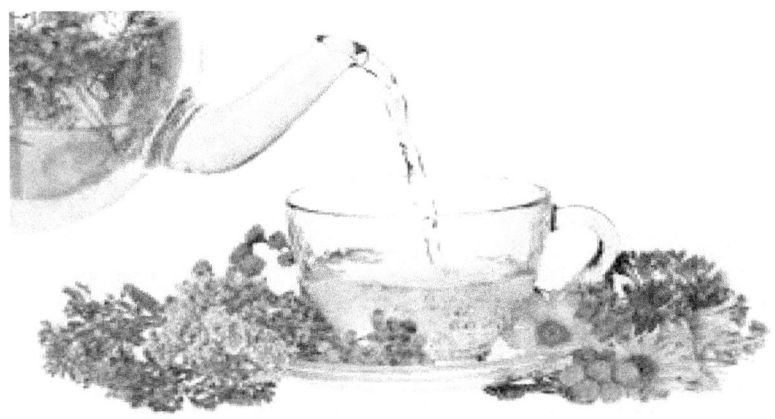

Health is the most important thing that every person is always concerned about, it is for the same reason that this eBook has been written. Check out chapter 4 to know the best nature's medicine for men and women. Have you tried all over the counter drugs to shed off the excess fats but nothing works? Look no further! Read chapter 5 to learn how fast you can lose the extra weight and reclaim back your shape. Read more to learn how you can lessen the number of trips you make to the doctor and use the medicinal plants in your backyard to improve your health condition.

Chapter 1: What Is Nature's Medicine

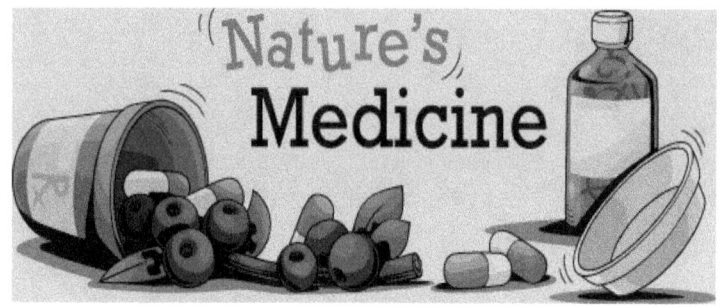

There is nothing abnormal with using the best natural medicine to treat different types of common illnesses. Vegetables, herbs as well as dried fruits have been known to cure common health problems for many years. These herbal remedies have been used by different cultures around the world until they were replaced by conventional drugs. However, health physicians are now advocating for these herbal medicines when treating long term illnesses.

Decades ago this was the best healing practice being used by many cultures around the world to treat the sick. However different communities used different types of plants. Over time healers learnt how to use different plants to cure the same disease. With time the practice has given rise to the science we use today, including chemistry, pharmacology and botany. There are two reasons why people prefer herbal remedies to the modern medicine practices.

First, modern medicine is a more about impersonal treatment, you just have to walk to a doctor's office, present your complaints to the doctor, then the doctor gives you a pill , what we do not know is that the pill we take does not solve the root cause of the problem. You go home thinking that everything is okay, only for the same health problem to start bothering you again. The second reason why people are opting to take herbal remedies, are the side effects that come with modern medicine pills. Just take some minutes to read the list of side effects and you will wonder whether the pill cures or causes more health problems.

Chapter 2: How Nature's Medicine Works

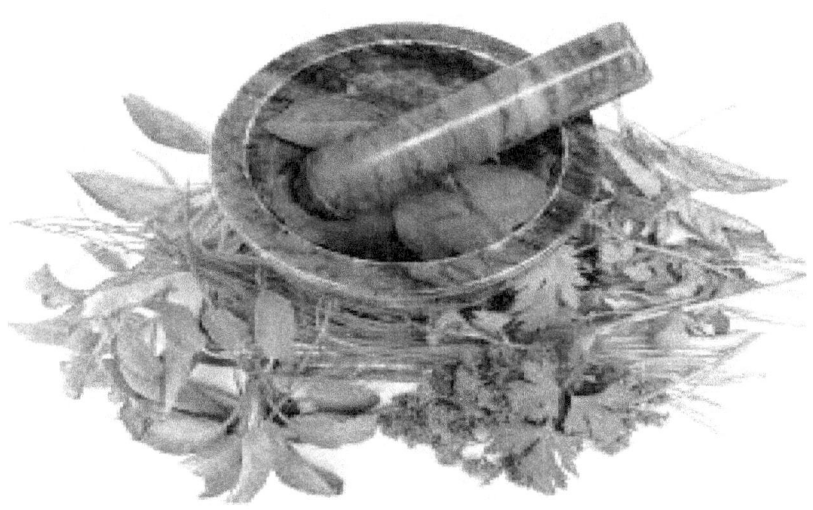

There are many ways in which herbal remedies differ from modern medicine techniques; they do not just address the symptoms, the treatment focuses on the root cause of the problem but not just a quick fix of the problem. The good news is that herbal remedies work with the natural body's immune system. Herbal medicine does not push foreign substances into your body and force them to work; rather it works with the body's immune system to fix the health problem without any side effects.

Most of the health issues we are facing today are because we have turned our backs on the health lifestyle. We eat unhealthy meals; we don't work out and breathe polluted air full of toxic chemicals. Isn't it obvious that we shall feel ill most of the time and end up running to the doctor? The pills we get from the doctors produce more common health problems. We must embrace new methods of treating ourselves so that we can stop having the same problem over and over again. One way through which we can take care of our health is by embracing the best lifestyles. Eat healthy, exercise every day, quit smoking, and have enough sleep.

Another reason you must use herbal remedies is because they help improve positive energy. As mentioned earlier they address the root cause of the health problem in your body/mind/ spirit making you feels much better because you don't have to worry about the side effects. It's because of its effectiveness that it has survived the test of time, and now more and more people have started realizing how helpful herbal medicine is to their lives. Natural medicine could be the healthiest way you can get healed without having to worry about the side effects.

Chapter 3: Most Common Natural Medicine for Men

Unfortunately, men do not like the idea of walking to an herbalist mainly because they do not like exposing their problems so that they cannot be thought of as weaklings. What these men do not know is all the health benefits they can get from herbs without having to live with the baggage of side effects resulting from modern medicine. There is no need to try to cure your current only to get some more complications, you can use the most sought after herbal supplements to stay more healthy and strong.

8 EFFECTIVE URINARY TRACT INFECTION HOME REMEDIES

1. Drink lots of Water
2. Eat Pineapple
3. Cranberry juice
4. Baking soda
5. Juices
6. Apple cider vinegar
7. Vitamin D
8. Probiotics

Natural remedies can help you in some many situations including prevention and treatment of the most common illnesses. Natural herbs can help avoid harsh prescription modern medicines that cause more problems than health. The good thing about herbal remedies is that they can help promote healing without forcing the body to heal unnaturally. Some of the most common health problems that men can solve using herbal remedies include prostate cancer, impotence, improving physical fitness and male menopause. In addition to the natural herbs, there are more vitamins and supplements that can help men deal with these issues.

There is no doubt that herbal medicine is what you should be looking for today, consider consulting a herbal specialist in case of any side effects. A herbalist can help you in case of allergic reactions or dosage amounts. Some of the herbs that you can use to address such health problems include red clovers, saw palmetto, ginkgo biloba, muira puama and American ginseng. Apart from the renowned herbal remedies, other ways in which men can improve their health naturally include:

1. **Proper exercise**: as old age kicks in our immune system it becomes weaker as the metabolism slows

down. As this happens we gain weight and this poses health problems such as hypertension, heart problems and diabetes. Exercising regularly while using natural herbs can greatly help to keep you in good shape and avoid long term illness such as diabetes and cancer.

2. **Diet**: someone once said, "we are what we eat " this goes hand in hand with exercises. The type of food we take greatly defines who we are, and things can get worse if we are not careful. You can use some of the best herbal remedies in tea or add them as spices to the food you take. You can contact your herbalist or research online in case you have some problems.

3. **Stress relief**: chamomile tea is one of the herbs that can help us relax. If used with other health techniques such as meditation, chamomile can help with the inevitable anxiety we face in our day to day lives. These are just a few of the remedies that you can use, as men grow old there are many health problems that come up , but you can get all over them if you consult a herbalist for the top notch herbal remedies.

Chapter 4: Nature's Medicine For Women

Natural herbs play a major role in women's health and healing. Just as there are special herbs that address male health problems, there are great herbal remedies that specifically cater for women health problems. A few years ago, these herbal remedies were used to treat mind and body health problems, but today they are becoming more widespread around the globe.

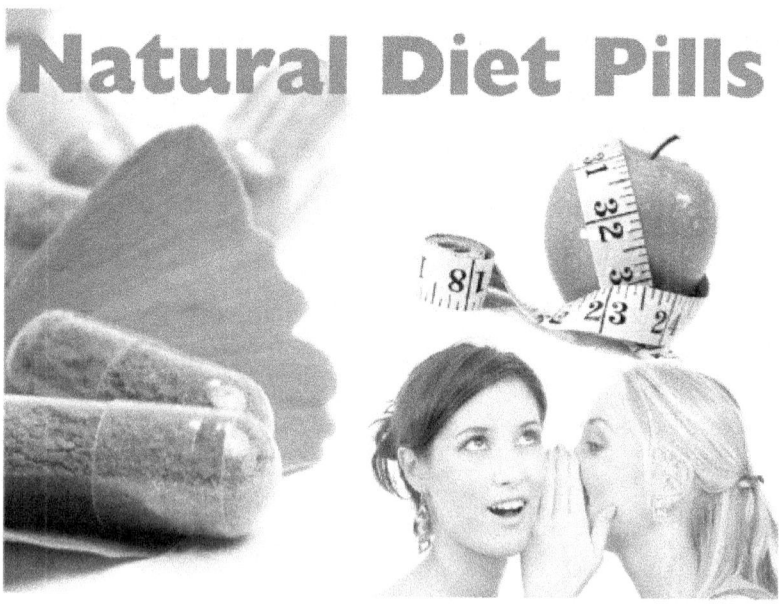

Natural Diet Pills

Why women should use herbal remedies

Statistics and research have proven that herbal medicine is a great alternative to the increasingly dangerous drugs that doctor's physicians prescribe. A doctor will prescribe the same drug over and over again even if it does not bring positive results. The main problem is that these modern medicines do more harm than good, and don't even address the disease they were supposed to target. The best natural herbs helps the body get back to its natural balance. Natural herbs are the best because they not only focus on the symptoms but they are also curative. Since they are natural, they do not have any side effects if taken as prescribed. Herbal medicine is also known to deal with several problems that affect women, including pregnancy, menopause, fertility and menstruation.

There are many mental and physical strains that come with pregnancy, but you don't have to worry any longer because there are great herbal roots that can help reduce the stress that comes when you are expectant. Most women think of the discomfort brought about by menopause as a disease, most end up on the doctors trying to get the best modern medicine that never works, to herbalists menopause is a natural occurrence and the only way to ease the discomfort is by using natural herbs. For many years women have been struggling with fertility issues with nothing to help in modern medicine, there are several herbs that can help with that. With the help of a herbalist, you will also be able to learn about natural herbs that can help ease the discomfort caused by cramps. There are many areas that natural herbs can help if well coupled with a proper sleep, stress relief, healthy diet and herbal supplements. Some of the natural herbs that can be used as health supplements include mugwort, nettle, mothwort, raspberry, cramp bark and black cahash. While there are many who might think of herbal medicine as an alternative to modern medicine techniques, time has come for nature to take its course in the healing process.

Chapter 5: Natures Medicine For Weight Loss

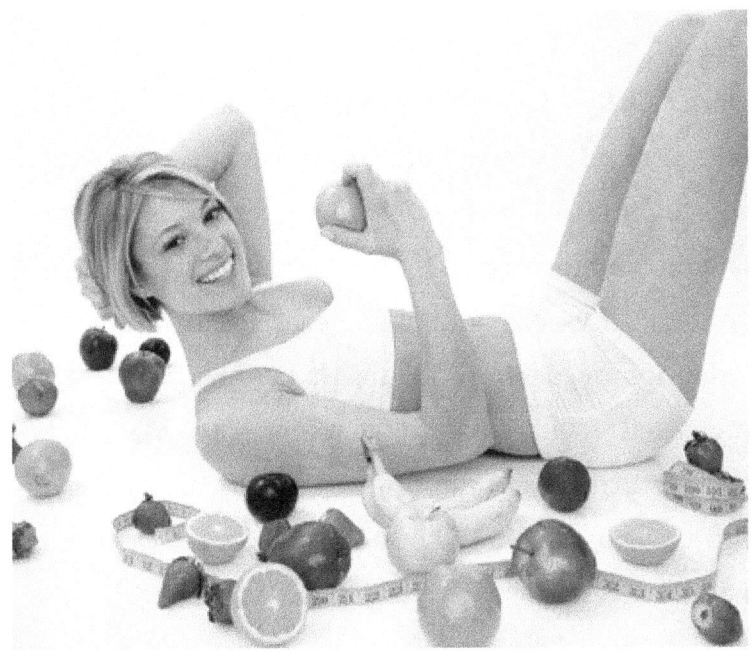

Today, there are many people using herbs to lose weight naturally. This has been for a while the safest and most effective way of losing weight in few days, with no side effects. You can easily boost your health by using natural herbs for weight loss without causing harm to your body. The latest research that has been conducted in the United States has shown that at least

1.7 billion people around the globe are obese. In the USA obesity is considered a disaster with over 65% of all the adult populace being overweight. 14% - 25% of children and teenagers are also suffering from this epidemic.

The rise in number of obese people in the United States can be associated with unhealthy eating habits, lack of exercise and stressful lives. In addition, over 500, 000 people die globally because of the weight related illnesses. Some of the worst health problems common among overweight people include stroke, gout, diabetes, hypertension, heart disease and cancer. Other minor health problems that come with increased weight gain are sleep apnea and osteoarthritis. The simplest way in which you can protect yourself from these illness is by embracing natural weight loss remedies.

Overweight individuals are more likely to suffer common health problems as compared to people who are within the right category. Proven herbal remedies help in weight reduction and this lowers the risks associated with obesity. According to professional physicians there are four things that a person can do to control their weight, they include strength training so that you can build up muscle, healthy eating taking note of the calories you take, cardiovascular exercise to increase metabolism and mental strength. Healthy eating includes taking the right herbal weight lose supplements such as bitter orange, cayenne, coleus, ephedra, garcinia cambogia, green tea, guarana, guggul, spirulina and St. Johns wort.

Keeping a journal can help control what you eat clearly outlining the calories present in the meal you have just taken. Seeing what you take during the day can greatly reduce the trips you make to the kitchen because you know very well the amount of calories you are supposed to take and what you have taken at that point will be more than enough. You cannot just lose weight by sitting around and waiting for it to happen, you must make informed decisions if you want to shed the extra fats. This can help embrace the best lifestyle suitable for natural weight loss techniques.

Chapter 6: Natures Medicine Remedies For Children

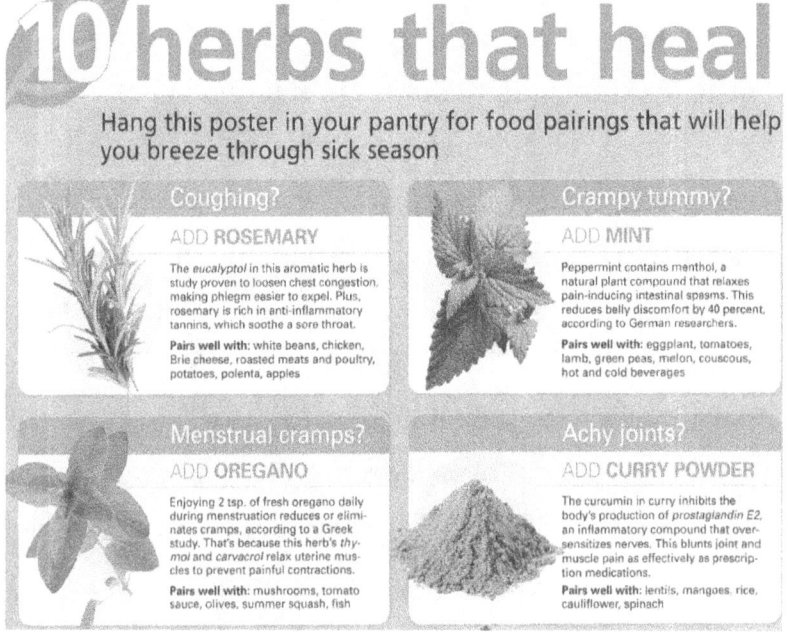

10 herbs that heal

Hang this poster in your pantry for food pairings that will help you breeze through sick season

Coughing?

ADD ROSEMARY

The *eucalyptol* in this aromatic herb is study proven to loosen chest congestion, making phlegm easier to expel. Plus, rosemary is rich in anti-inflammatory tannins, which soothe a sore throat.

Pairs well with: white beans, chicken, Brie cheese, roasted meats and poultry, potatoes, polenta, apples

Crampy tummy?

ADD MINT

Peppermint contains menthol, a natural plant compound that relaxes pain-inducing intestinal spasms. This reduces belly discomfort by 40 percent, according to German researchers.

Pairs well with: eggplant, tomatoes, lamb, green peas, melon, couscous, hot and cold beverages

Menstrual cramps?

ADD OREGANO

Enjoying 2 tsp. of fresh oregano daily during menstruation reduces or eliminates cramps, according to a Greek study. That's because this herb's *thymol* and *carvacrol* relax uterine muscles to prevent painful contractions.

Pairs well with: mushrooms, tomato sauce, olives, summer squash, fish

Achy joints?

ADD CURRY POWDER

The curcumin in curry inhibits the body's production of *prostaglandin E2*, an inflammatory compound that over-sensitizes nerves. This blunts joint and muscle pain as effectively as prescription medications.

Pairs well with: lentils, mangoes, rice, cauliflower, spinach

There is evidence that natural medicine can help cure little children completely. Fortunately, most parents have realized this and are taking their children's to qualified herbalists when they start developing health problems. The most common illness in small children includes sore throat, flu's and stomachaches. Instead of buying over the counter drugs, parents can use the best herbal remedies to address these illnesses.

Today, you will find natural medicine on supermarkets and drug stores, but most parents ignore them because they don't know what to buy. On the other hand, dieticians who focus on children are not able to give the right advice because they don't understand how natural medicine works. What you should know is, natural herbs have been in use for many years, they have also been tested and proven to be perfect for restoring children's health. Keep reading to learn about the most effective herbal remedies that can help resolve your kid's illnesses.

1. **Stomachaches/Upset Stomach**

Ginger is a great herb that stimulates secretion of gastric juice, saliva and bile juice. It is also believed to tone up peristalsis; recently clinical trials have also shown that ginger can alleviate pregnancy discomforts such as nausea and vomiting. The good news is that ginger is easily available; you can always have it in hand by keeping it in a freezer. Herbalists say that kids can chew or drink ginger tea to calm vomiting. In addition, ginger roots can be put in hot water, and then added to a mango juice to make it smooth for children.

Chamomile tea has also been proven to be safe for children suffering from cholic; it also calms an upset stomach. Health experts have shown that its anti-inflammatory properties help relax the intestinal walls minimizing stomachaches and cramping. Peppermint tea can also help calm down an upset stomach in babies. Statistics have also shown that children who took peppermint tea had significant reduced stomach pains compared to those who took modern drugs such as placebo.

2. **Diarrhea**

Constant diarrhea flushes out important bacteria, but you don't have to worry about that anymore because probiotics replenishes the healthful bacteria and restores good health in the intestines and hence slows down diarrhea. The good news is that probiotics is easily available and is common in several foods. When eaten they helps the body build immunity to a number of diseases and illnesses. Yogurt is also an important addition to a kid's diet because it helps reduce the diarrhea duration in children. Research has also shown that peppermint oil helps boost cramping, diarrhea and constipation symptoms associated with bowel syndrome. Parents can use prunes or other dried fruits which are natural sources of fiber, by mixing them into cereal. Also remember to give your child lots of water so that their body can be able to absorb the fiber. You should also encourage your kids to participate in exercise and workouts because they can greatly stimulate bowel movements and increase metabolism.

3. Mild Burns

While many people think that aloe Vera is the best herbal remedy for cooling and soothing the skin, tamanu oil is the most effective natural medicine to sooth a kid after burns. Tamanu oil is known to form a scar tissue that improves healing, this helps the burned skin to grow and heal much faster. You can also try out the extracts of witch hazel tree for faster results after a burn. The good news is that it is commonly available in medicated pads, ointments and as a liquid in drug stores. Health experts have tested and found out that witch hazel has a great protective effect.

4. Fever

Ginger tea root is the best herbal remedy for low grade fever illness in children. The antimicrobial properties of ginger root are what make it a good prescription choice. In addition, ginger is able to eliminate the rhinovirus that causes cold in small children. All you have to do is to take a ginger root, put it in water and then boil and give the concoction to your child.

5. Bruises

Arnica gel or cream is the best solution for inflammation and bruising in kids. You can easily get the arnica gel from the arnica flower. It's a great component to have in your medicine rack because it reduces swelling and bruising faster and efficiently. In addition, subsequent lab tests have shown that arnica gel has anti- inflammatory and anti –microbial affects. Experts have also said that arnica cream relives osteoarthritis hence reducing joint swelling and pain. Other studies have proven that arnica gel helps reduce bruising much faster compared to vitamin k placebo ointments. All what you have to do is visit your nearest drug store and ask for the arnica gel, follow the instructions and you will see how amazing it is when it comes to quick and effective healing.

6. Allergies

Allergic children can greatly benefit from eating natural honey made by bees; environmental allergies such as pollen grains, dust, grass and many more should not trouble your child any more. Nevertheless, parents should never give honey to children under one year. Study has shown that honey made by local bees is a source of clostridium botulinium spores that causes infant botulism and very serious intestinal condition. Bacteria present in the clostridium botulinium spores can easily multiply producing dangerous toxins in baby's gastrointestinal tract. Another good natural remedy for allergies is the saline nose spray which reduces irritation and swelling caused by allergic responses. You can easily make the solution at home, boil water, let it cool to room temperature and add table spoon, then put the solution in a spray bottle, your child can then squirt the solution into the nostril.

7. **Sore Throat**

You can easily cure a sore throat in a day or two, by using apple cider vinegar mixed with a tablespoon of local honey coupled with 6 glasses of water a day, until the symptoms disappear. Cider vinegar kills and soothes the bacteria's present in your throat. If possible you should ignore the honey, but use it to make the solution palatable because it can be rough. Honey makes it sweeter and eases the roughness.

8. **Colds**

To heal cold, herbalists believe that nothing works as efficiently as chicken soup. Experimental results have shown that chicken soup contains anti-inflammatory effects and can alleviate cold in small children. However, parents should avoid buying chicken soup with low sodium levels because it's the salt effect present in the chicken broth that reduces swelling and inflammation. You can buy and then frozen it so that it will always be available in your house whenever your kids need it.

Chapter 7: Nature's Medicine /Modern Conventional Techniques

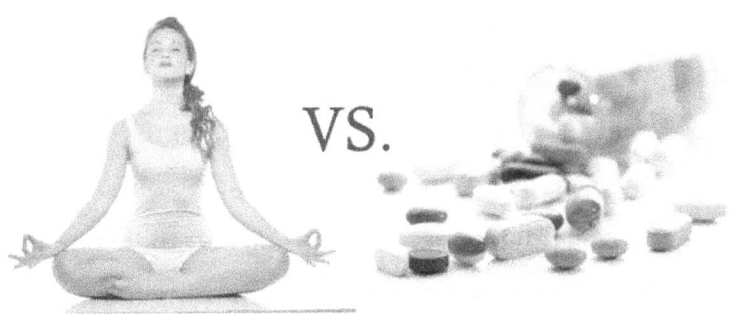

Today, there are two types of medicine to choose from when you are feeling unwell. Modern conventional techniques prescribe drugs that restrain the immune system causing lethal side effects. However, conventional drugs work perfectly well when it comes to emergencies and surgical operations. On the other hand, natural medicine which is more affordable addresses the root cause of the health problem and brings positive results. Natural medicine focuses on prevention and resolving the underlying condition once and for all, rather than just addressing the symptoms. Natural medicine treats and restores the immune system helping the person to recover much faster.

What Is Conventional Medicine?

People, who rely on conventional medicine, visit the doctor's office when they are ill looking for treatment. They don't think that there are better ways in which they can prevent the health imbalances before the disease develops. Basically, conventional medicine defines health, as a state where the body works perfectly without signs of any disease. Herbalists consider this as a negative way at searching for health problems. As a matter of fact there are lots of differences in regard to how herbal and conventional health experts define health.

Natural medicine does not just focus on the disease symptoms, its aim is to create a health balance in your body by relieving the symptoms and prevent future illnesses. Herbal medicine helps make your body immune system much stronger improving its capacity to fight disease in days to come. You should be patient because natural medicine does not deliver instant results. It may even take longer than you had anticipated in case your body's immune system was at the verge of breaking down. Natural medicine takes a much gentle approach to cure the body from the inside out. On the other hand, conventional medicine is known for a more aggressive treatment approach using terms such as "quick fixes" to describe their drugs. There is no doubt that everyone wants a magic bullet, but it could be better if there were no lethal side effects to cope with.

Cost Of Treatment

Most people are more concerned about health, safety and effectiveness of the treatment rather than the cost. Whether it's over the counter drugs, herbs or food the more effective it is towards addressing your health problems the better. Currently, many people are turning to herbal medicine because they know it does not come with side effects and is less expensive. Statistician has shown that more people living in the United States have been forced to skip prescription drugs because of the high costs. This means that you can save much by choosing to buy the more affordable natural medicine.

Regulation Of Herbal Medicine And Drugs

The food and drug administration monitors the safety of pharmaceutical drugs, most people have been duped into thinking that FDA tests the drugs themselves but that is not true. The drug company only submits their tests results and FDA proves that the drugs are 100% safe. There are many health experts who believe that this practice could be biased in favor of the drug companies. On the other hand, herbal remedies are regulated by FDA as food and not drugs. As a result, herbal manufactures have been given the sole responsibility of ensuring that their cures are safe, without having to register their herbs with the FDA.

The only exception where the herbal supplement manufacturers are required to submit their product samples to the FDA is if the ingredients have just been newly introduced in the USA market. Nature's medicine manufacturing companies use FDA perfect manufacturing procedures to make sure their ingredients meet top notch quality standards. However, the FDA is responsible for making sure that the herbal cures are perfect, and should take action against the manufacturing company whenever side effects are reported.

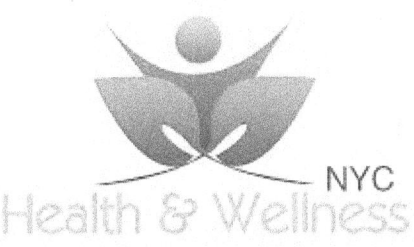

Today, natural medicine is more popular than ever before. People have realized how helpful these herbal remedies are when it comes to improving their general health and leading healthy lifestyles. There are over 100 studies that have shown amazing benefits of countless herbs and herbal gels. Research has proven beyond reasonable doubt that regularly taking herbal supplements coupled with a healthy lifestyle can help lead a long healthy life free from illnesses.

Chapter 8: 4 Ways To Relive Pain Using Natural Medicine

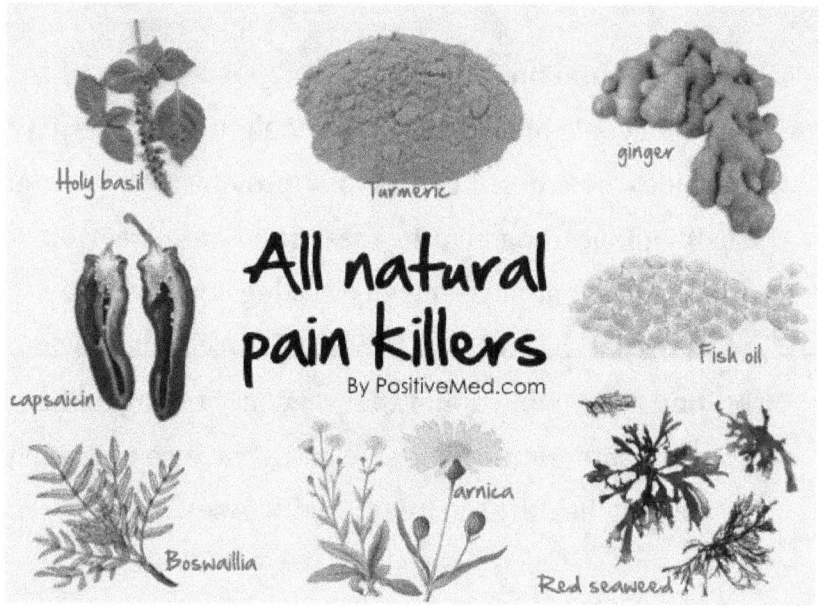

Holy basil

Turmeric

ginger

All natural pain killers
By PositiveMed.com

Fish oil

capsaicin

Boswaillia

arnica

Red seaweed

Are you feeling lots of pain to an extent you think that old age has come earlier? You can easily turn to herbal medicine to relive the pain without any side effects; there are several herbs that you can use to reduce the pain from head to toe. While herbs can strengthen your immune system and treat illness, you should contact a health physician before you start taking any herbs to avoid adverse side effects. For instance, a person who is just about to undergo a surgical operation should not take ginger or turmeric because they are widely known as blood thinners. If you suffer from arthritis and chronic pain, chances are that you have some pills in hand, or you toughen up. Today health professionals are turning to natural pain relief natural remedies such as yoga or acupuncture. As a matter of fact, pain is one of the reasons why many USA citizens are turning to alternative medicine.

1. Eucomnia For Back Aches

Herbalists use eucomnia tree backs to alleviate joint and back ache. Eucomnia is also used to strengthen bones, ligaments and tendons. Eucomnia helps heal tissues that have been weakened by constant stress. Studies have shown that eucomnia leaves and bark contains an element that speeds up the development of collagen. While it can be used alone, herbalist strongly suggests it to be used alongside other herbs. A word of caution, adults taking hypertension drugs should consult a physician before taking eucomnia or any other supportive herbs.

2. Valerian Root

Also referred to as a natural tranquilizer, valerian root greatly relieves pain if well used. It has been used by herbalists for many years to relieve insomnia, anxiety, irritability, stress and control the nervous system. It is also used to reduce pain because it reduces the sensitivity in nerves. You don't have to continue taking ibuprofen for pain relief, just give a cup of valerian a try and you will be thrilled to see how fast and effectively it works.

3. Ginger Treats Nausea And Stomach Aches

Ginger roots have been used for decades to cure pain because of its anti-inflammatory effects. Some of the health problems that ginger cures include menstrual cramps, headaches, arthritis and joint pain. Surprisingly ginger can also be used during winter because its boosts blood circulation. As perfect addition to biscuits, sweets, vegetables and tea ginger can be used in any way, as long as it lands in your stomach. Just cut the ginger root, boil for 10 minutes and drink as tea. You can also alleviate the pain by applying the ginger concoction to the affected areas. Take a cloth, put it in hot water for 30 seconds, and then let it cool before placing it on the affected area for 30 minutes.

4. Use Turmeric To Calm Pain

Turmeric, a great herb used in curry powder has great pain relief benefits. Studies have shown that turmeric has anti inflammatory and cancer properties that boost blood circulation, it also prevents blood clotting. For a while now, turmeric has been used to ease pain in bruises, sprains, strains and relives joint inflammation. Turmeric can also help treat digestive and skin problems. Turmeric contains curcumin to reduce the number of enzymes that causes inflammation. All you have to do is to put a spoonful of turmeric powder when cooking.

Chapter 9: Using Natural Medicine To Boost Your Immune System

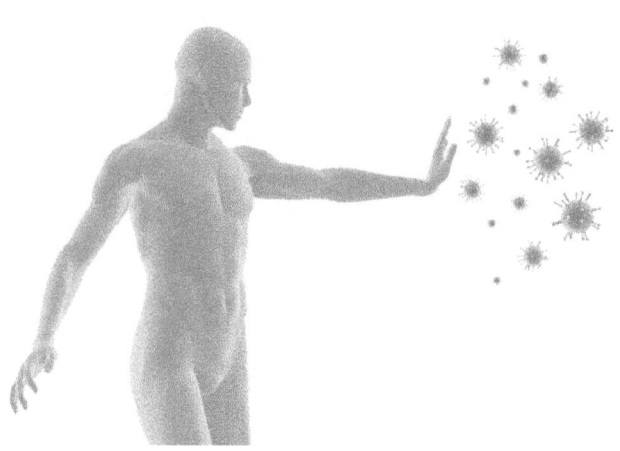

A strong immune system is a huge benefit to everyone who is concerned about his/her health condition. During winter many people opt to go for vitamin c or flu shots as preventive measures, so that their children don't fall sick and skip classes and also to keep them in the right state of health. What many people fail to realize is the fact that boosting your immune system has many more benefits not just about preventing flu and colds. Natural health supplements works perfectly well to prevent other diseases and immune disorders, and helps you live a long healthy life.

Most of us have a weak immune system because of the lifestyle choices we make. Today, everyone is busy looking for more cash and this puts much stress to our bodies and minds. As a result very few people remember to take care of their bodies. Our suggestion is that you should not let emotional stress, anxiety, insomnia or poor eating habits lead you astray from boosting your immune system. Keep in mind that a weakened immune system makes your body venerable to many health issues from bacterial to viral and fungal infections. Worse, a weak immune system makes you an easy target for cancer because it's not able to fight off foreign cancerous cells. Don't forget that toxins and chemicals will have lethal effects if you have a weak immune system. Improving your immune system prevents your body cells from ageing prematurely.

What Are The Benefits Of A Strong Immune System?

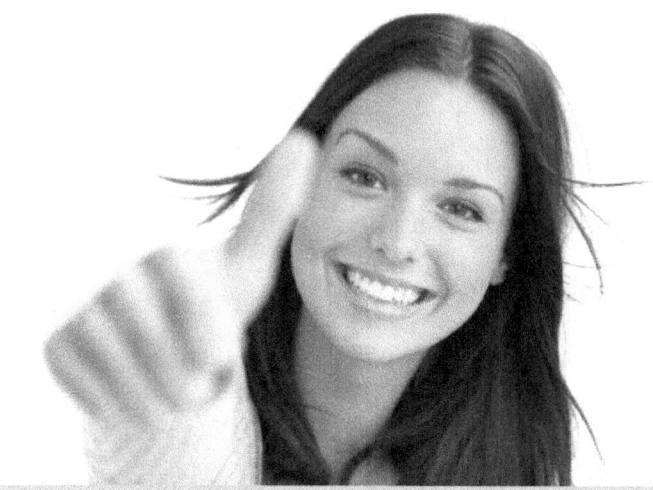

Strong Immune System

Most people think that the immune system is a single entity, but that is not the case. This is a system and requires balance for it to work harmoniously. Boosting your immune system is noble given that it provides your body with many health benefits. In addition, you don't have to take prescription drugs because your body will be able to effectively fight off any foreign bodies. Basically, your immune system treats your body with natural supplements, this way your body will be full of energy to keep off foreign substances. A strong immune system helps cure your affected body cells and reduce the effects of again, it also fights off toxic substances, defends your body against bacterial and viral infections. All these benefits can help lengthen your life, improve your stamina and energy levels and in great health.

Ways In Which You Can Boost Your Immune System

Our poor lifestyle and eating habits are the root causes of a weak immune system, changing what you eat and the way you live can greatly change and strengthen your immune system. Check out some of the things you can do to improve your immune system and lead a healthier lifestyle.

a. **Eat healthy:** poor healthy eating habits are one of the biggest causes of a weak immune system. A diet rich in fruits, vegetables, whole grain and proteins can greatly boost your immune system and enhance your energy levels. Apart from a smooth digestive process, drinking plenty of water can really help enhance your immune system.

b. **Exercise**: regular exercises boost the cell effectiveness and mobilize your immune system to fight infections. A five minute walk can also help boost your immune system if you don't have enough time to work out in the gym. In addition, this is the cheapest way of boosting your immune system because you don't have to pay anything for it.

c. **Shed excess fats**: obesity restrains your body's systems from functioning properly including the immune system. Keeping your weight in check can really help in strengthening your immune system and keeping in shape.

d. **Get enough sleep**: I understand that we are living busy lifestyles, waking up as early as 3am so that we can be able to pay the bills, ignoring the fact that our bodies need enough rest. Straining our brains /bodies to work excessively without getting enough sleep at night weakens our immune system. Enough sleep at night for at least 8 hours can really improve the way our immune system works.

e. **Change your lifestyle**: do you smoke, nicotine weakens your immune system and the only way you can boost it, is by quitting. You also need to stop drinking or lessen the amount of alcohol you take. If possible, eliminate alcohol from your drinking list completely. You should also be keen to avoid any chemical toxins in your place of work or at home. Substances such as industrial fumes weaken our immune system and affect the way it functions. Remember to read labels on food containers because of the lethal risk factors. Most importantly avoid cigarette smoke at all cost, because smoking is the most significant threat to the immune system.

How To Boost Your Immune System Naturally

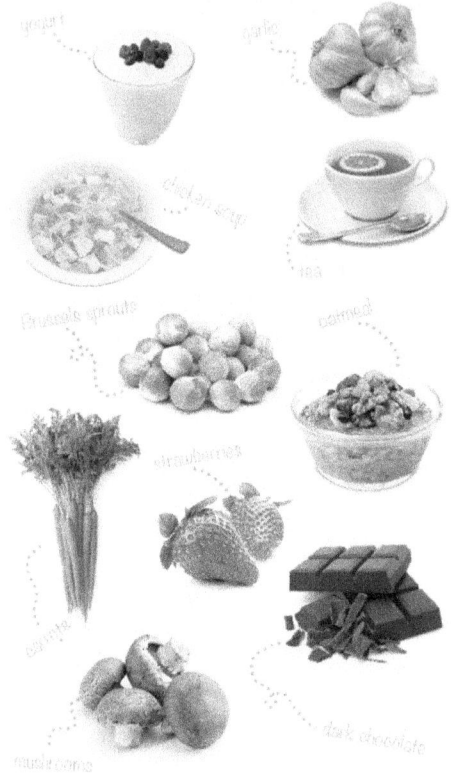

Apart from eating healthy foods, minerals (zinc and selenium) and vitamins can also help boost the immune system. You don't have to worry about this if you have been eating healthy. Some of the natural vitamin supplements that can really help in boosting your immune systems include vitamin c and e. Other benefits of using herbal immune supplements include better blood circulation, enhanced liver function, healthier immune system and improved cell health.

Chapter 10: Heath Benefits Of Natural Medicine

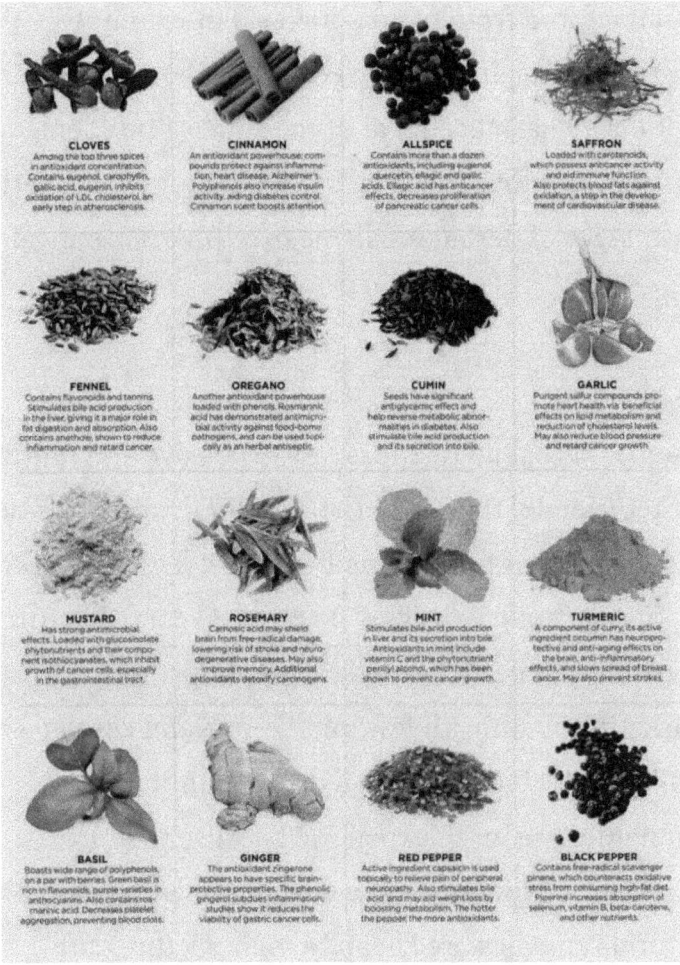

While the scientific study of herbal medicine is very new, there are many known benefits of nature's medicine. You should consider the merits of herbal medicine before you make the difficult decision of taking them. Despite the fact that herbal medicine is facing lots of negative criticism from conventional health experts, it's important to remember that most of the pharmaceutical drugs you find today are manufactured from plant sources. For example, aspirin was originally derived from willow bark, digitalis a pharmaceutical drug for heart problems was derived from foxglove flowers. Read more to learn the advantages of herbal medicine over pharmaceutical drugs.

Cheap: herbal medicine is less expensive and more pocket friendly than over the counter drugs. Statistics has proven that natural medicine cost less compared to pharmaceutical drugs. The reduced cost of natures medicine can be attributed to testing, a short marketing chain with few middlemen and ease in availability. Pharmaceutical drugs manufactured companies are more expensive because they are processed and marketed as a commercial product. Natural remedies are cheap to manufacture and produce.

Ease in availability: finding the right type of herbal remedy for your illness is quite easy because they are made from spices, herbs, fruits and vegetables.

Decades ago people used to grow medicinal plants in their backyards and it was much easier to find the right herbal remedies. Today, most people live in urban areas where there is no enough space and can only get medicinal plants, fruits and vegetables in local supermarkets. Just visit your local supermarket and look for lemon, honey, ginger, garlic, apple or thyme and you will be amazed by the great medicinal benefits that come with these products. Herbs are locally available without a doctor's prescription; as a matter of fact you can grow herbs such as chamomile or peppermint in your backyard.

Fewer side effects: most nature's medicines do not have any lethal side effects than conventional medicines so it can be perfect to use for long term results. There is no doubt that pharmaceutical drugs contain effective ingredients that help cure illnesses, but its effects do not stop there. Over the counter drugs affect your immune systems functioning with their lethal side effects. The most common side effects being nausea, vomiting and drowsiness. These side effects will be a thing of the past if you start using homemade nature's medicines.

Effectiveness: Nature's medicine tends to have a long term health effect than pharmaceutical drugs because they treat the root cause of the health problem, but not the symptoms. In addition, herbal remedies treat several minor illnesses at the same time. Ginger or honey can treat a wide range of illnesses including stings, pimples, arthritis, bad breath, athlete's feet, acne scars, bruises, sinus, leg cramps, constipation, weak memory, peptic ulcers, mouth ulcers, obesity, tired eyes, warts, yeast infection, water retention, headache, ear infection and many more.

Clean: natures medicines are manufactured from the same ingredients that we use in our kitchens in our day to day lives, you can rest assured that herbs are clean by using them according to the instructions provided by a health expert. Compared to pharmaceutical drugs that are made differently, you are 100% aware of the way herbal medicines are made and nothing should make you think that they are unclean. In addition, natural herbal remedies are fresh and unspoiled. This makes it easier for them to target and cure the illness fast and effectively. Keep in mind that herbal remedies have few or no side effects at all.

Conclusion

Everyone who reads the contents of this book understands clearly what he/she must do to strengthen their immune system or lose weight without having to visit a health physician. I strongly believe that you will be able to reclaim back your health after reading this book given that herbal remedies are also easy to find. The information outlined in this book address the common health problems that people are facing on daily basis. Whether its obesity, arthritis, sore throat or heart disease you will be able to learn the right herbs that you can use to get better.

With the help of this eBook, parents will find effective herbs that they can give their children so that they can strengthen their immune system and become healthier. To make it easier for people without medical knowledge to understand, the book has been written using the simplest terms possible. Everything that you needed regarding natures medicine has been well demonstrated from chapter xx to xx. That said you should consult a herbalist for more information regarding natures medicine. It should be much easier for you to get all the herbs listed on this book because they are locally available in supermarkets.

www.ingramcontent.com/pod-product-compliance
Lightning Source LLC
Chambersburg PA
CBHW070506290526
45790CB00003B/1111